D1232872

Understanding tinnitus – managing the noises in your ears or in your head

Keith Dunmore
Glynis Riddiford
Valerie Tait

Published by RNID

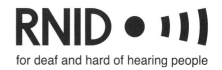

RNID ● ❙❙❘

for deaf and hard of hearing people

Published by RNID
19-23 Featherstone Street
London EC1Y 8SL
Tel: 020 7296 8000
Textphone: 020 7296 8001
Fax: 020 7296 8199
E-mail: information@rnid.org.uk
Website: www.rnid.org.uk

ISBN 1-904296-02-5

Picture acknowledgements:
Front cover: Rich Reid/National Geographic/Getty Images
Pages 29-31: Medical Photography. Addensbrookes Hospital
Pages 10-11: Gillian Lee Illustrations

Design by RNID Publications
Edited by Gill Kirby

Introduction

We would like to thank the patients and audiology staff at Chase Farm Hospital who helped with this book. All the names of patients who shared their experience of tinnitus with us have been changed.

About the writers

Three health care professionals have written this book. They all have experience of working with people with tinnitus and have all had tinnitus themselves.

Keith Dunmore

Keith started his career in audiology in 1979 as a student audiologist. In 1988 he became chief audiologist and head of audiology at Peterborough's new Edith Cavell Hospital. In 1999 he undertook a part-time MSc at University College London. In 2001 he took up his present post at Chase Farm Hospital, where he is audiology service manager/senior chief audiologist. Keith is a member of the British Association of AudiologisTs and British Society of Audiology.

Glynis Riddiford

Glynis has a degree in Education Studies. Her work with children with disabilities, particularly children with communication and hearing difficulties, led her into hearing therapy in 1997. She now works at Chase Farm Hospital where she is involved in providing a comprehensive tinnitus management service. This includes a course on relaxation. In 1999 Glynis trained at Birmingham School of Audiology to teach relaxation to patients who have tinnitus.

Val Tait

Val has a degree in English Language and Literature and was a teacher for many years. Her increasing hearing loss gave her the opportunity to change direction and she has been a lipreading teacher and hearing therapist for eight years. Val currently works at Chase Farm Hospital where she is deputy audiology services manager and head of hearing therapy. She comes from several generations of deaf people. As a freelance writer she also writes a regular column for RNID's magazine *One in Seven*.

We would also like to thank those people who gave us valuable feedback about the book, especially Gerhard Andersson, Don McFerran, Catherene McKinney and Catriona Williamson.

Gerhard Andersson

Gerhard has a PhD in both clinical psychology and otorhinolaryngology. He has worked in the field of tinnitus for the last 12 years and is currently a clinician and researcher at the University of Uppsala, Sweden. His research includes cognitive behaviour therapy, brain imaging, psychopathology and cognitive aspects of tinnitus. He has written extensively on tinnitus and has had a book published on tinnitus.

Don McFerran

Don is a Consultant Otolayrngologist in Colchester, Essex. His interest in tinnitus began in the late 1980s when he worked with Jonathan Hazell at the Middlesex Hospital.

Catherene McKinney

Catherene has been working in the field of tinnitus since 1990. She currently heads the Audiology department at Guy's and St Thomas' Hospital NHS Trust. She also runs a tinnitus and hyperacusis clinic at the Portland Hospital. She has completed extensive research into the effects of habituation management for tinnitus.

Catriona Williamson

Catriona has been managing the RNID Tinnitus Helpline since 2002. Prior to this she worked as a hearing therapist in Cambridge and Nottingham. She has been working with people with tinnitus for the last 10 years.

About this book

If you think you might have tinnitus, or have just been diagnosed as having tinnitus, this book will help you understand more about your condition. We also tell you more about where to go for help and support, and about the kind of help you can get on the NHS.

Most people find that tinnitus improves over time, even if they do nothing about it. However, you can do many things about tinnitus and this book tells you about some of them. You will find many suggestions that have helped a wide range of people. Everyone is different, so not everything will work for you, but none of these suggestions will work unless you try them. We have also included stories from people who have learnt to manage tinnitus.

Reading a book is not a substitute for seeing a specialist.
If you are worried about your tinnitus you should visit your GP (your local doctor). They should refer you to the nearest ear, nose and throat (ENT) department. From here you may also be referred on to a special tinnitus clinic if there is one in your area.

This book is written for adults with tinnitus. However, many of the strategies described in this book will also help children. If your child has tinnitus, or you think they may have tinnitus, speak to your GP. You can also contact the British Tinnitus Association for more information. See *Chapter seven* for contact details.

Foreword by
Dr Ewart Davies

I am delighted to write a foreword for what is an excellent treatise of tinnitus. The book clears the many misconceptions that are held about tinnitus and I hope that it will be well read by both medical and audiological professionals as well as people with tinnitus. It provides invaluable and concise information about the widespread incidence of the condition, and where to get help and advice, as well as details of the equipment and therapy that is available to help manage the condition. It also presents advice on relaxation therapy, stress prevention and sleep maintenance, all important factors in the treatment of tinnitus. It is outstanding in the way it presents unbiased opinions of the different factors that influence tinnitus perception and the potential of different therapeutic regimes.

Dr Ewart Davies has recently retired from the Department of Pharmacology at the University of Birmingham Medical School. Much of his research revolved around the investigation of the mechanisms that give rise to tinnitus, and the testing of drugs and other agents that may help tinnitus. His interest in tinnitus persists and he now spends much of his time as Chairman of the British Tinnitus Association and encouraging research into the condition.

Contents

Chapter one
What is tinnitus?

This chapter aims to help you begin to understand more about tinnitus. It looks at:

- What we mean by tinnitus.
- What it sounds like and how it affects different people.
- Some of the known causes.
- Theories about tinnitus.

What do we mean by tinnitus?

Tinnitus is a medical term for any noise which people hear in one ear, both ears or in their head. These sounds do not come from outside the head, although they may occasionally sound as if they do. Apart from one or two rare conditions, tinnitus cannot be heard by anyone other than the person who has it.

What does tinnitus sound like?

Tinnitus sounds can take a variety of forms, such as buzzing, ringing, whistling, hissing, or a range of other sounds. For some people it can even sound like music. Sometimes people only notice these sounds when it is very quiet, such as at night. Other people find that they are much louder and can intrude on everyday life. Sometimes tinnitus noise beats in time with your pulse – this is known as pulsatile tinnitus.

This is how some people have described their tinnitus:

"Like a plane engine."

"A ringing which is worse in the morning."

"A slight rushing which I only hear when it is quiet."

"Exactly like a generator in my right ear."

"A bee buzzing."

"Tuning fork in my left ear."

"A slight rustling."

"Like a cricket."

"Constant drone of different noises."

What is it like to have tinnitus?

The effect that tinnitus has on different people can vary tremendously. Whilst most people are not bothered by their tinnitus, others find that it has a serious effect on the quality of their lives.

People often think that tinnitus is a sign of serious illness, although this is rarely the case. They may assume that they will develop a hearing loss as a result of tinnitus – whilst tinnitus can be associated with hearing loss, many people with tinnitus have normal hearing. Some people find tinnitus quite frightening. They worry that it will get louder, or go on forever, or that they will never be able to enjoy complete silence again. They may find that reactions from friends, family or medical professionals can be quite negative, which can make them feel worse. Some blame themselves, or even someone else, for their tinnitus, which in turn makes them feel guilty or angry. These are all very normal reactions. People with tinnitus often find they also have sleep problems, which usually improve as their tinnitus gets better. See *Chapter four* for more information.

"When I first heard my tinnitus I was quite frightened because I didn't know what it was and I imagined all kinds of horrible things. My tinnitus sounds like a rushing noise, which is more noticeable to the right where I get a whistling noise as well. It is worse when I am tired or stressed, those things definitely play a part."

"I worried and worried, my husband worried too... some people at work had had tinnitus and said such things about it that I became quite frightened... they really scared me."

People are often most affected by tinnitus when they first get it and it can make them very stressed. The stress makes their tinnitus worse, which in turn makes them more stressed - a vicious circle.

It is important to remember that help is available and with time you will learn to understand and manage tinnitus.

"My tinnitus is much better now. I don't hear it at all when I'm busy. It doesn't bother me any more. I've got my life back."

"The tinnitus is much better. I hardly give it a thought. I don't think about it unless someone asks me how it is. I have no problems sleeping or anything."

How common is tinnitus?

Most people have experienced brief periods of tinnitus at some time or another. It is quite common to have it for a short while after you have been exposed to loud noise. Tinnitus is very common in people of all ages and so it's important to realise that you are not alone.

In 1987 the MRC Institute of Hearing Research based in Nottingham carried out a study into the prevalence of tinnitus.

They found that:

- 10% of adults have had tinnitus for longer than five minutes.
- 7% of adults have been to see a GP about their tinnitus.
- 4% of adults have tinnitus that annoys them moderately or severely.
- 1% of adults have had tinnitus that severely affects their quality of life.
- 0.5% of adults have tinnitus that affects their ability to lead a normal life.

What do we know about tinnitus?

In 1953 two researchers called Heller and Bergman put a group of young, healthy students in a soundproof room. None of them had tinnitus. They were then asked to record what they could hear. Although none of them could hear any external sounds, nearly all of them reported hearing sounds and noises – sounds which were the same as those reported by people with tinnitus. This shows that in the right environment many people can experience the sound of tinnitus.

Why do some people get tinnitus?

It is important to remember that tinnitus is a symptom and not a disease. There are many different causes of tinnitus. We do know that tinnitus can be linked to exposure to loud noise, hearing loss, ear or head injuries, some diseases of the ear, ear infections or emotional stress. It can also be a side effect of medication, or a combination of any of these things. We explore some of these causes below.

However many people with tinnitus have never experienced any of the above and don't have a hearing loss. There are several theories and ongoing research as to what happens when you have tinnitus.

Some of the known causes of tinnitus include:

Ear infections

If you have an ear infection it can cause discomfort and tinnitus and may lead to hearing loss, especially if it is left untreated. It is important to visit your GP, who will be able to treat the infection.

Noise exposure

There is a lot of evidence to connect continued exposure to noise with hearing loss and tinnitus. Loud sounds can damage your hearing, especially if you listen to them for hours at a time. Try to avoid them at home and when you go out. Make sure your workplace follows the Noise at Work regulations to limit the amount of noise you are exposed to at work. You can contact the RNID Tinnitus Helpline for more information about noise exposure and how to protect your hearing.

Stress

Most people have some stress in their lives. It is almost unavoidable. While stress does not directly cause tinnitus, it can make it worse. Many things can cause stress. A significant period of stress or a significant stressful event, such as the death of a close relative, has been known to trigger tinnitus.

Your tinnitus itself may be making you feel stressed. That is why stress management is an important part of tinnitus management. By learning to relax and take control you can help your body and brain manage tinnitus. We look at what you can do to manage stress in *Chapter three*.

Circulation/blood disorders

There are several main blood vessels that pass close to the ear. Normally you do not notice the blood flowing through these. Occasionally, if you have a medical condition that affects your circulation, such as thickening of the arteries or anaemia, it can disturb the blood flow and you might start to hear it. It is unusual for this to happen. This sort of tinnitus is often known as 'pulsatile' because it sounds like the heartbeat. High blood pressure can make it worse. Some of the causes of pulsatile tinnitus can be treated medically or you may be shown techniques to help you manage it.

Respiratory, muscular and other noises
The body cannot function in total silence. Just as you can sometimes hear the blood in your veins and arteries, you might also be able to hear other normal bodily functions. This may be due to breathing or movements of the muscles, especially those around the head and neck.

Drugs
Your GP will be able to talk to you about any possible side effects of drugs you have been prescribed. Drugs that may be damaging to the ear or hearing are known as ototoxic. There are very few ototoxic drugs. They are rarely prescribed and then only to patients ill in hospital. In many cases these drugs are prescribed to save your life and this is likely to outweigh the risk of any side effects. You should also be strictly monitored when you are prescribed ototoxic drugs.

Some people with tinnitus think that it was caused by, or has been made worse by, a medicine they have been prescribed. Although a large number of drugs list tinnitus as a possible side effect not everyone will develop tinnitus as a result of taking that drug. This is partly due to the way that the side effects of drugs are reported but also because we all react differently to drugs. Even though a drug may make someone else's tinnitus worse it may not have the same effect on *your* tinnitus.

It is also worth remembering that your tinnitus may not have been caused, or made worse by, the drug you are taking. It could just be a coincidence that this appears to have happened at the same time that you started taking the drug. The condition that you have been prescribed medicine for may also be making your tinnitus worse, rather than the drug you are taking for it, particularly if your condition is making you anxious or stressed.

If you are concerned that a drug you have been prescribed is making your tinnitus worse you can discuss this with your GP. You can ask about an alternative drug, which does not list tinnitus as a side effect. If you start taking a new drug and it makes your tinnitus worse, ask your GP if you could take a different drug. Sometimes you will need to continue taking the drug even if it is making your tinnitus worse, as there may not be any alternative available.

Below we have listed some of the common drugs reported to cause, or make, tinnitus worse:

- **Antimalarial drugs** – such as quinine and chloroquinine. These are prescribed to prevent you getting malaria or to treat malaria. Although these can cause permanent damage to hearing when taken in high doses, there is no evidence of permanent damage when taken in the low doses that are prescribed for malaria. They can give some people temporary tinnitus. If you are planning to travel to a malaria-infected area you **must talk** to your GP, or practice nurse, about taking antimalarial drugs.

- **Anti-inflammatories** – taken to reduce swelling.

- Some **antidepressants** – used to treat depression.

- Some **antihistamines** – taken to prevent or reduce allergic reactions.

- Some **antihypertensives** – taken to reduce high blood pressure.

- Some **diuretics**. Diuretics, or 'water tablets' are commonly used to treat high blood pressure. The small doses used are unlikely to cause tinnitus. However, some diuretics are used in much larger doses to treat conditions such as kidney failure, and these doses can occasionally cause tinnitus.

- **Aspirin**. Aspirin is taken to relieve pain, reduce fever and is used in many medicines for colds, period pain, headaches and joint or muscular pains. It also helps blood clots from forming. It contains salicylate, which is an ototoxic drug.

If you already have tinnitus you may find that even a small dose of aspirin may make it worse. This does not happen to everyone and you may find taking a single tablet has very little effect, but some people are more sensitive to aspirin than others. If you do think aspirin is making your tinnitus worse, speak to your GP to see whether an alternative medicine would be more suitable, particularly if you are taking aspirin as a painkiller. The effect of aspirin on tinnitus is usually reversible, which should mean that when you stop taking aspirin your tinnitus should return to its previous level. However, aspirin may cause tinnitus to last for longer if you take it over a long period of time or in higher doses.

You should *not* alter the dose of any medication you are taking, or stop taking it as a result of reading this book, unless the GP who prescribed the medication agrees it is safe to do so. If you have any questions about any medication you are taking, or are about to take, speak to your GP or pharmacist.

Menière's disease
Menière's disease is a very rare, progressive condition of the inner ear. The underlying cause is unknown. People with Menière's disease have bouts or episodes of the condition, which include tinnitus, dizziness and fluctuating hearing loss. This is separated by periods when they are not affected by it at all – known as remission.

It is important to speak to your GP about this condition. They will refer you to an ear, nose and throat (ENT) specialist at your local hospital.

Ear syringing
Some people have occasionally reported that they have developed tinnitus after ear syringing. This is not common and it is even more unusual for syringing to do real damage to the ears. However, if you are worried about having your ears syringed, discuss it with your GP. There are other ways to remove wax using microscopes, suction apparatus and tiny instruments.

Your GP may have to refer you to an ear, nose and throat (ENT) department for this sort of treatment.

Understanding how your ear works

It is important to remember that the majority of tinnitus is not due to physical causes. To understand what happens when you have tinnitus when there is no obvious physical cause, you first of all need to understand how your ears work.

Our ears have three sections: the outer ear, the middle ear and the inner ear.

The outer ear

The outer ear consists of the pinna, which is the part you can see on the side of your head, and the external auditory canal (ear canal), which is the passage that sound travels along. This canal is about 2.5cm long and lined with skin. If you look at someone's ear from the side, you can see the entrance to it.

The part of the canal near the outside has hairs, and glands that produce wax. Together these keep it clean. The eardrum – the tympanic membrane – covers the other end of the canal. When sound reaches the eardrum from the outside it vibrates. Beyond the eardrum is the middle ear.

The middle ear

The middle ear is a space or cavity about 1.3cm across, filled with air. The cavity is connected with your nose and throat by the Eustachian tube. Most of the time the tube is closed, but if you yawn, swallow or blow your nose, it opens. You may notice a clicking sound in your ear when this happens – this is normal.

Between the middle ear and the inner ear is a wall of bone, which has two small openings in it, the oval window and the round window, each sealed by a membrane.

The ear

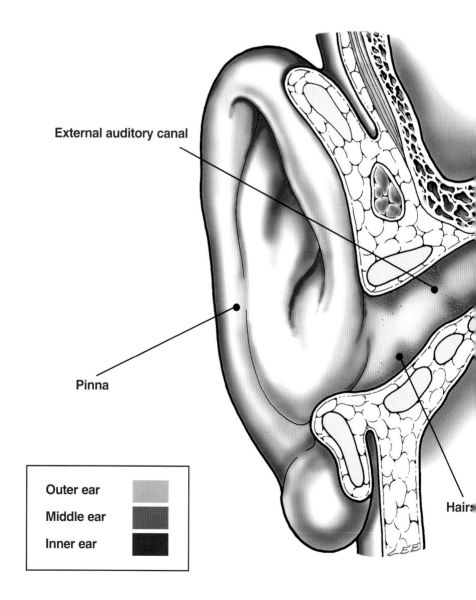

External auditory canal

Pinna

Outer ear

Middle ear

Inner ear

Hairs

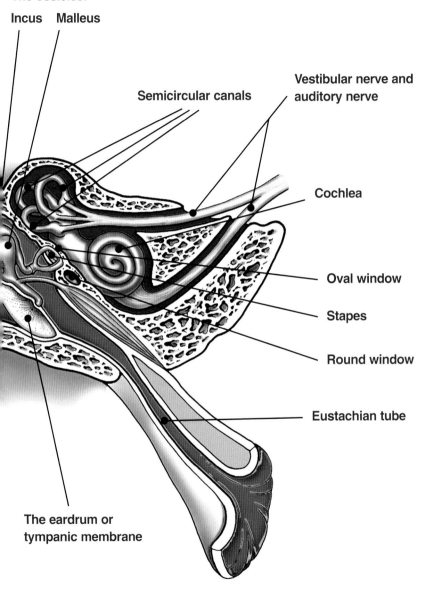

The ossicles:

Incus Malleus

Semicircular canals

Vestibular nerve and auditory nerve

Cochlea

Oval window

Stapes

Round window

Eustachian tube

The eardrum or tympanic membrane

A chain of three tiny bones stretches right across the middle ear cavity to conduct sound from the eardrum to the oval window. These three bones, the ossicles, are called the malleus, the incus and the stapes. They are also sometimes known as the hammer, anvil and stirrup.

The malleus is attached to the inner side of the eardrum, the incus stretches between the malleus and the stapes, and the base of the stapes fits into the oval window. When sound enters your ears and makes the eardrum vibrate, the vibrations pass from the eardrum along the ossicles. The stapes pushes like a little piston against the membrane in the oval window. Behind the oval window is the inner ear.

The inner ear

The inner ear has two parts – the cochlea and the semicircular canals. Both are embedded in bone.

The cochlea

The cochlea – the hearing part – is a spiral tube about 3.5cm long which coils 2.7 times. The spiral contains two fluid-filled chambers – an outer and an inner one. The outer chamber starts at the oval window, continues to the tip of the cochlea and then doubles back, ending at the round window. The vibrations caused by sound pass from the stapes through the oval window and into the fluid in the outer chamber.

The inner central chamber of the cochlea contains the Organ of Corti. This has about 17,000 small hair cells arranged in rows along the length of the cochlea. The hair cells have tiny rows of muscle protein on the upper surface – these are the 'hairs'. They are not real hairs, but when seen under a powerful electron microscope they look like hairs, hence the name. The under side of each hair cell is connected to nerve fibres which join other similar fibres to form the auditory nerve (also called the acoustic nerve, cochlear nerve or nerve of hearing). This goes from the cochlea to the brain.

When sound waves enter the fluid of the cochlea, they move the tiny hairs, causing the hair cells to send electrical messages to the auditory nerve. Different frequencies of sound are picked up by different hair cells, depending where they are located in the spiral tube. The nerve passes impulses up to your brain, which recognises them as different sounds – for example, people talking, or footsteps.

The semicircular canals
The semicircular canals are not used for hearing – they are part of your balance system. They are filled with fluid and have hair cells, rather like those in the cochlea. When you turn your head, the fluid in the canals moves and the tiny hairs on the nerve endings bend. Nerve impulses travel to your brain along the vestibular nerve, giving information about the direction your head is moving in.

The mechanics of tinnitus
The reasons why some people get tinnitus when there is no obvious cause are complex and are still being researched. There are several different 'models' or schools of thought as to how tinnitus is produced and experienced. Current views are that tinnitus is the result of the complex workings of several of the body's systems. These can all work together to produce what is experienced as tinnitus.

The hearing pathway has a complex filtering system which allows you to 'tune in' to sounds that have meaning to you, and 'filter out' sounds which are not important to you. This system works all the time and stops you being bombarded with sound. Your brain also has response systems that respond to the meaning of sound and help influence the way that you filter sound. Together these filters and response systems help to control how you react to sound. For example, if you hear your name at a party you will tune in to hear what is being said about you. This is because the sound of your name has lots of meaning to you.

Your hearing pathway, your filters, and your sound response systems are all involved when you hear tinnitus. Firstly, a tinnitus signal is present, usually in your inner ear or the auditory nerve but it could be anywhere in the hearing pathway. This is usually very weak and most people don't notice it. However, if you become aware of tinnitus, this means that your filters have started to pick up this tinnitus signal. If you become anxious or annoyed by your tinnitus then your sound response systems will tune your filters into your tinnitus and you will start to hear it more. The good news is that your filters and sound response systems can be taught to ignore the tinnitus signal – this process is called 'habituation'.

When you get professional help for your tinnitus your therapist may prefer a particular school of thought and will treat you based on that model. Although there are various schools of thought none of them claim to be the only effective way to treat tinnitus. We tell you more about getting help for your tinnitus in *Chapter three*.

Is there a link between sensitivity to sound and tinnitus?
Around half of people with tinnitus are also more sensitive than normal to everyday sounds. Broadly speaking there are two forms of sensitivity to sound:

Hyperacusis
If you have hyperacusis you may find everyday sounds uncomfortable or painfully loud, even when they do not bother other people.

Misophonia/noise annoyance
If you have misophonia, also known as noise annoyance, you may find particular sounds extremely irritating, although you may not be particularly sensitive to sounds in general. If your dislike is strong enough to be considered a phobia then the term phonophobia is used.

Hyperacusis and misophonia can be treated with habituation therapy and sound therapy. We tell you more about these later.

Measuring deafness and hearing loss

In this book you will find that we use specific terms to describe deafness and hearing loss – normal, mild, moderate, severe and profound. These are specific terms used by audiologists and we have provided a brief explanation of those terms below.

Deafness and hearing loss are usually measured in units called dBHL – dB stands for 'decibels' and HL stands for 'hearing level'. A hearing test finds the softest sounds a person can hear – their thresholds – across a range of frequencies (pitches of sounds). The greater the threshold level – in dBHL – the greater the hearing loss.

- Anyone with thresholds between 0 and 20 dBHL across all the frequencies is considered to fall within the range of 'normal' hearing.

- People with mild deafness have some difficulty following speech, mainly in noisy situations. The quietest sounds they can hear fall between 21 and 39 dBHL.

- People with moderate deafness have difficulty following speech without a hearing aid. The quietest sounds they can hear fall between 40 and 69 dBHL.

- People with severe deafness rely a lot on lipreading, even with a hearing aid. British Sign Language (BSL) may be their first or preferred language. The quietest sounds they can hear fall between 70 and 94 dBHL.

- People who are profoundly deaf may communicate by lipreading and/or BSL. BSL may be their first or preferred language, however, severely or profoundly deaf adults, who became deaf later in life, rarely use BSL. The quietest sounds they can hear in their better ear average 95 dBHL or more.

Some people may have the same hearing loss in each ear, or it may be different in each ear.

Deafness and hearing loss are usually measured in units called dBHL

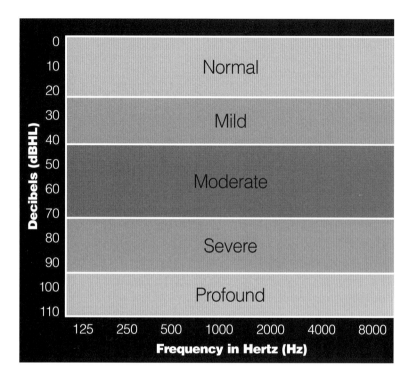

Chapter two
Getting help for your tinnitus

If you have tinnitus, or would like to learn more about it, there are lots of different ways you can find out more and get help. This chapter looks at:

- How to contact professionals who deal with tinnitus.
- What sort of professional help you can expect to get.
- How to find out more yourself.

Remember, you can always take a friend, relative or partner with you to any appointments you have. They can help you remember what you were told about tinnitus, ask questions and raise concerns of their own. If they understand about tinnitus it can help them to give you support.

Getting professional advice

Most people who are troubled by tinnitus would rather seek expert help than just read about it. This is very sensible and there are two main ways of doing this in the UK.

- Private clinics.
- The National Health Service (NHS).

Getting help privately

Many consultants divide their time working between the NHS and private clinics, so you may well see the same people whichever option you choose. With private treatment you have more of a choice about when you see a consultant, and where, but you will of course have to pay and you may have to travel further to see them.

If you decide to consult a tinnitus expert privately you will find that different clinics have different arrangements for patients to be 'referred' to them. You will need to consult your GP first to get a referral. Most tinnitus experts will only take referrals from an ear, nose and throat (ENT) consultant or audiological physician – this could be someone you have seen privately or via the NHS. If you have private health insurance, it is sensible to check first to find out if it will cover treatment for tinnitus and what kind of treatment.

If you do not have private health insurance it is important to find out the cost of the consultation with the doctor and the cost of further investigations, such as hearing tests and scans, as well as the cost of any tinnitus therapy the consultant may recommend.

Getting help on the NHS

The NHS service varies depending on where you live. Some areas have specialist tinnitus centres or clinics in their hospitals. Some areas may offer a limited tinnitus service, or in some cases, no tinnitus service at all. Your local hospital will be able to let you know about the services it provides and the RNID Tinnitus Helpline can tell you about services across the country. Getting an NHS appointment may sometimes involve delays and waiting lists, so be prepared to wait.

Contacting your GP

The first person you will need to see is your GP. They will be able to check that your ears are free from wax and infection and make a suitable referral to the ENT department at the hospital. Although GPs are trained to a high level in a wide area of medicine they are not tinnitus experts and their knowledge about treatment for tinnitus may vary.

Unfortunately when some people visit their GP about tinnitus they are still told, "you'll have to learn to live with it", and find it difficult to get a referral to an ENT department. Make sure you tell your doctor that your tinnitus is a problem and how it is affecting you – for example, is it making you feel stressed, or giving you sleep problems? Are you finding it difficult to cope with? It may be useful to take along some leaflets about tinnitus. You can get hold of free copies from RNID or the BTA. It can also be very helpful to take along a friend or relative as well.

If you still cannot get a referral try seeing a different doctor in the practice or even changing to a different practice altogether. You do have the right to a second opinion.

Fortunately most GPs are helpful and it is worth seeking their help:

"My GP was very helpful and as soon as he heard what the problem was he referred me at once."

"The first person I turned to was my GP. He thought I had an ear infection and gave me antibiotics. When they didn't work he sent me to a specialist. My GP has been very helpful and encouraging."

What will happen at the hospital?
At the hospital you will first see a specialist at the ear, nose and throat (ENT) department. Staff in the audiology department will also see you, as this is generally where you will be treated for tinnitus. It is important to have a thorough check-up to see if there are any obvious causes for your tinnitus. You may then be referred to a tinnitus clinic if there is one in your area.

Ear, nose and throat departments (ENT)

The staff in the ENT department are all medically qualified. They will look into the cause of your tinnitus by taking a medical history and examining you. To help them to make an accurate diagnosis they may refer you to the audiology department for tests.

Audiology department

The staff in this department will be able to give you tests for tinnitus (diagnostic tests) as well as show you how to manage it (rehabilitation). You will meet different staff depending on the size and set-up of the department and you might meet more than one person. These include:

Audiologists/Audiological scientists

These two professions are very similar and their duties often overlap. They deal with both diagnostic testing and rehabilitation. They are responsible for testing your hearing and, if necessary, fitting a hearing aid. Many people find that a hearing aid can help their tinnitus, but not everyone. They may also offer tinnitus counselling and help with balance problems.

Hearing therapists

Hearing therapists help rehabilitate adults with:

- An acquired hearing loss (a hearing loss that you have developed later in life rather than one you were born with) and/or
- Tinnitus and
- Sometimes balance problems.

They will take you through a tinnitus management programme and monitor your progress. If your hospital does not have a hearing therapist the audiologist will usually provide this service.

Clinical psychologists

These are not based in audiology departments and not all audiology departments are able to refer people to them. Tinnitus can lead to stress and anxiety. Some people blame many of their problems on tinnitus. Clinical psychologists can help you become less stressed and gain a balanced view of your tinnitus. They often use a technique called cognitive behavioural therapy. This is based on the idea that people can change how they think and behave. We give you more information about cognitive behavioural therapy in *Chapter three*.

What happens at a typical hospital appointment?

Different clinics and hospitals are set up in different ways, however, the following is a typical scenario.

When you first arrive at the hospital, you will be asked to check in at the ENT reception in the outpatients' department.

In the consulting room

The ENT consultant, or one of their medical staff, will take a medical history. This will take the form of a series of questions about your general health and more specific questions about your hearing, balance and tinnitus. They will then examine your ears. After this, they will send you for some diagnostic tests in the audiology department.

Diagnostic tests

The audiologist, or audiological scientist, will carry out various tests to see how well you can hear and whether you have any problems in the middle ear. The tests will vary but may include the following:

Audiogram

This involves listening to a series of pure tones or 'whistles' through headphones, while sitting in a soundproof room. A hearing test finds the softest sounds you can hear – your thresholds – across a range of frequencies (pitches of sounds). The greater the threshold level, the greater the hearing loss. From your response to these sounds, the audiologist will be able to plot your hearing threshold across a range of frequencies, from low to high tones. This is called an audiogram.

Tympanogram

For this test you will be asked to sit still for around 10 to 30 seconds. A small probe will be placed in your ear. A machine will measure how well the eardrum, muscles and bones in your middle ear are working.

Tinnitus match (pitch and matching)

Some ENT departments will also try to identify the exact pitch and loudness of your tinnitus. This is done by producing a tone and asking you if your tinnitus is higher or lower than the tone. After you have responded, the tone is altered. The process is repeated until the pitch of your tinnitus has been identified. A similar test is done to find out how loud your tinnitus is. There is some debate about the usefulness of these tests.

Back to the consulting room – explanation of tests

After these tests you will see the same member of the medical team that you first saw. They will then decide if you need more specialised tests, or whether they have enough information to make a diagnosis. If they make a diagnosis they will either treat the condition causing the tinnitus or refer you back to the audiology department for a course in tinnitus management. You can find more information about tinnitus management in *Chapter three*.

If you do need further tests they may include:

Auditory brainstem response (ABR)

This test measures the electrical signal produced by your ear in response to sound as the signal travels along the nerve into your brain. Three sticky pads will be placed on your head – one on your forehead, or on the top of your head, and one by each ear. You will then be asked to listen to some clicks through headphones while a machine measures your response.

Magnetic resonance imaging (MRI)

An MRI scan is similar to an X-ray because it shows details of what is happening under your skin. Unlike an X-ray, it can also show details of your nervous system and can take a picture of a cross section of your ear. This gives the consultant lots of detailed information.

Computerised tomography (CT)

This is a specialised computerised X-ray that is sometimes used instead of an MRI scan.

If you do need any of these tests, they are normally performed during a separate hospital visit and you may have to wait a while before you can have them. After you have had the tests, you will be given another appointment to attend ENT outpatients when the specialist will explain the results and discuss the options available to you.

How to find out more yourself

Tinnitus information services

There are a number of information services that deal with health issues, including tinnitus. You can find full contact details about these services in *Chapter seven*.

RNID Tinnitus Helpline

You can contact the RNID Tinnitus Helpline by telephone, textphone, e-mail, fax or letter. The Helpline can provide the following information for people with tinnitus and their friends and families:

- Support and general advice for those with tinnitus or their family and friends.
- Free factsheets, leaflets and other information about tinnitus.
- Books and relaxing CDs and cassettes you can buy.
- Contact numbers of useful organisations.

- Contact details of support groups and self-help groups.
- Details of your nearest hospital-based tinnitus clinics.
- Details of the latest research on tinnitus.

British Tinnitus Association (BTA)

You can contact the BTA Helpline for information, advice and support by telephone, e-mail, fax or letter. The BTA:

- Campaigns for better services for people with tinnitus.
- Supports a network of local tinnitus groups around the country.
- Has a range of publications and produces a quarterly magazine, *Quiet*.

The BTA can give you:

- Details of local self-help groups.
- Details of your nearest hospital tinnitus clinics.

NHS Direct

NHS Direct can provide information about a wide variety of medical conditions, including tinnitus. The people answering your call are trained healthcare professionals. They can provide basic information about tinnitus and some of its causes. You can also access NHS Direct on the Internet.

Self-help books

Many books have been published over the years about tinnitus and its treatment. These can be very helpful. You should remember though that one person's experience can be very different from another's. Some books are written by non-professional people, writing about their own experiences and tinnitus management techniques. Their insights into tinnitus can be extremely valuable. Other books are written by health care professionals, who have spent much time and research on their work. Always look at the writer's qualifications, experience and motivation before deciding which books to read.

We've included a list of suggested books in the *Further reading* section at the end of this book, but your ENT or audiology department may be able to recommend some other titles.

Internet

You will find a lot of information about tinnitus on the Internet and much of it is excellent. However, as with books, never believe everything you read on the Internet, but make an informed decision. To help you decide, try and find out:

- Whether the person or organisation that has created the website is qualified to comment on tinnitus.

- How much research they have done.

- Whether they are writing about something that just works for them, or does proper medical evidence back up their information?

- If they work with people who have tinnitus, or they have just 'read up' about it?

- Who has created the site and why? Has it been set up by someone who has tinnitus, so that they can share information about the relief and help they got? Has it been created by a health care specialist, who has devoted much time, effort and research to tinnitus management and who wants to share the results of this with the public?

- If the site is trying to sell something, look at the site's claims and the research behind these claims. Don't necessarily be put off. Some of the world's leading tinnitus experts run private clinics and have excellent websites full of very valuable information.

We have included a list of informative tinnitus websites in *Chapter seven*. You can also contact the RNID Tinnitus Helpline for suggestions of useful websites.

Denise's story

Denise has a severe hearing loss and tinnitus in her right ear.

I went to my doctor because I had this continuous buzzing noise in my right ear. My family pushed me into doing something about it and finding out about the problem. I was saying "pardon" all the time and trying to lipread half the time. The tinnitus was always there and it got worse gradually. I was straining to hear with my good ear. At night it was dreadful – it sounded like a generator.

My GP did tests and sent me to the hearing clinic. The doctor at the hospital said I'd had a bad virus, which had damaged the nerves in the right ear so that I'd lost a lot of hearing and got the noise as well.

I saw the hearing therapist and we talked about me having a hearing aid. She said that hearing aids not only helped deafness, they also helped tinnitus.* I was so desperate with the noise that I decided to give it a try. The lady at the audiology department, the audiologist, adjusted the hearing aid to suit me and I could hear much better and the tinnitus is not nearly so prominent. It's much lighter and doesn't worry me so much at all. They put the hearing aid in my bad ear. As I say, the tinnitus is much better. I hardly give it a thought. I don't think about it unless someone asks me how it is. I have no problems sleeping or anything and I can hear beautifully. It just shows what a difference a hearing aid makes.

*Although hearing aids can be helpful for many people with tinnitus they will not help everyone. You can find out more about how hearing aids can help tinnitus in the next chapter.

Chapter three
Managing tinnitus

This chapter looks at the different ways you can start to manage your tinnitus, including management techniques available from professionals and ways you can start to help yourself.

What is habituation therapy?

Although there is no cure for tinnitus that works in the same way for everyone, it is occasionally possible to treat the underlying condition that may be causing tinnitus and there are ways to manage it. Habituation therapy works by changing your sound response systems so that you gradually become less aware of the tinnitus (you can find more information about your sound response systems in *Chapter one*). Habituation therapy can involve:

- Hearing aid(s).
- Sound therapy, including using a sound generator.
- Relaxation therapy.
- Counselling.

Habituation usually takes from six months to two years. It is not a quick fix but happens gradually. Some people find that, over time, their tinnitus goes away or they stop being aware of it. Others find that although it is still present in some circumstances, it becomes much less intrusive.

You may find that different audiology departments use slightly different methods to help you habituate to tinnitus, but they all tend to use a combination of the following.

Hearing aids

If you have a hearing loss, using a hearing aid may help tinnitus. The audiologist will discuss the different options and styles of hearing aids that are available, including whether you need one or two hearing aids. All NHS hearing aids and batteries are provided free of charge.

A hearing aid can help with tinnitus management by:

- Helping to compensate for your hearing loss.
- Stopping your ears straining to hear.
- Increasing the information available to the brain by picking up background sounds around you. All these will help distract you from paying attention to tinnitus.

Not everyone finds that a hearing aid helps tinnitus. Contact the RNID Tinnitus Helpline for more information about hearing aids.

Sound therapy

Sound therapy is also known as 'sound enrichment'. Many people find that they are more aware of tinnitus in a quiet environment. Sound therapy works by filling the silence with therapeutic sounds. These distract you from listening to tinnitus and so make it less noticeable. It also helps reduce the contrast between the tinnitus and background sounds, so making the tinnitus appear less intrusive. This helps your 'filters' to tune out tinnitus. Sound therapy involves listening to a range of sounds that you find pleasant, such as recordings of the sea or a woodland glade, the TV, music, a sound generator, or a sound enricher. Sound therapy can be used in many situations – for example, during a daily relaxation session, at bedtime, or while driving.

Sound generator

If you do not have a hearing loss, a sound generator may help (this is also known as a white noise generator or a wide band sound or noise generator). This produces a gentle, soft 'rush' (white noise) which sounds like an off tune, or off station, radio. This can help retrain your brain to ignore tinnitus. The volume should be set at just below the level of the tinnitus. You can get different styles of sound generator. You may not be offered all styles on the NHS as availability varies throughout the country. It will also depend on what is most appropriate for your needs:

You wear an **in-the-ear sound generator** in the outer ear. It is small, easy to 'pop in' and you do not need an ear mould. However, because they are not custom-made they may not fit your ear very well. The controls are rather small and fiddly so they are not ideal for people with sight or dexterity problems. They can be worn in bed, although you may find them uncomfortable if you lie on your side, and so they suit people whose tinnitus affects them during the day or night. However, you may prefer to try some of the sound generators designed specifically to be used in bed (see below). In-the-ear sound generators are not suitable for some people as they can block off natural sounds around you and affect your hearing.

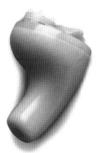

In the ear sound generators are easy to put in

A **behind-the-ear sound generator** looks like a behind-the-ear hearing aid. You will need to wear a custom-made earmould. An audiologist will take an impression of your ear so that an

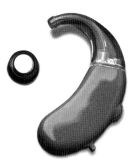

You should wear a behind-the-ear sound generator during the day

earmould can be made. Once this has been done, you will be invited back to see a hearing therapist who will explain how to use the sound generator. You should wear it during the day, usually for a minimum of six hours, and it therefore suits people whose tinnitus is more noticeable during the day. It is not designed to be worn in bed. Behind-the-ear generators do not tend to affect your hearing as they can be worn on an 'open-mould' so that you can hear natural sounds around you. They are therefore ideal for people with normal hearing.

An **under-the-pillow sound generator** is a little box that goes under your pillow so that you can use it at night. It is not designed to be worn in, or behind, the ear. You can either programme it to stay on all the time or set the time switch which means that it will switch itself off after a period of time. If you wake during the night and are bothered by your tinnitus, you can turn it back on again.

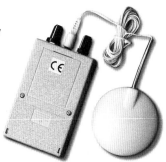

An under-the-pillow sound generator is a box that goes under your pillow at night

You can use a **bedside sound generator** beside your bed or anywhere in the home or office. They are often called sound enrichers. As well as white noise they often produce other sounds such as waves, fountains, rain and birds. They are useful for anyone needing help with their tinnitus, day or night. Some people like to use them during a relaxation session. You can get both battery or mains powered models. Again, they can play continuously or you can set them to turn off automatically after a period of time.

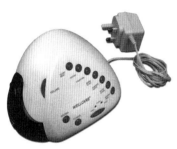

You can use a bedside sound generator beside your bed or anywhere in the home

A **sound pillow** looks like a normal pillow but it has two speakers inside it. You can connect these to your radio or stereo to listen to sounds of your choice at night. Alternatively you can get **under-the-pillow speakers**, that you can connect to your stereo, or bedside sound generator, and then place under your pillow.

You may be able to get under-the-pillow and bedside sound generators on the NHS. You can also buy them privately. The RNID Tinnitus Helpline can give you details of current suppliers.

A sound pillow looks like a normal pillow

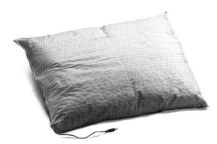

31

You can connect under-the-pillow speakers to your stereo

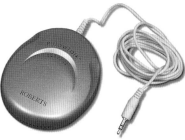

You can also get combined hearing aid/sound generators. These are not widely available on the NHS but your local audiology department will be able to advise you and discuss whether they are suitable for your needs.

Remember that a sound generator will only help you if you use it when you are advised to. The sound from a sound generator should be softer than the sound of your tinnitus. It should also be a neutral sound and most people will not be aware of it after a period of time. The hearing therapist or audiologist will give you all the advice you need.

Hyperacusis

People with hyperacusis can become very sensitive to sound. This can mean they avoid sound as much as possible, even going so far as to wear earplugs or earmuffs. This only makes hyperacusis worse. If you have hyperacusis (see *Chapter one*) sound therapy can help train your brain to become less sensitive to sounds. Your audiologist will work out an individual habituation programme with you and discuss how best to manage this condition. However, treatment usually involves using a sound generator set at a very low volume to begin with. The volume is gradually increased over a period of time until you are able to tolerate normal sound. It is then returned to a lower level.

Household sounds

Some people find normal everyday sounds helpful, such as the television, the radio, a ticking clock, an electric fan, or the shower. You should be careful not to cover the sound of tinnitus by playing these sounds too loudly.

Music

Many people find that listening to classical music works better than listening to 'pop music'. 'Easy listening' music may also help. Ideally the music should be neutral and again, be careful not to cover the sound of tinnitus by playing it too loudly. People with tinnitus have recommended baroque and Gregorian plainsong chants but you may have to experiment until you find the sort of music which works best for you.

Natural sounds

If you look in your local high street shops, you will often find a selection of 'new age' cassettes, CDs and videos. These contain natural sounds, such as the sea, dolphins, the rainforest or birds, either on their own or combined with pleasant music. These are enjoyable, relaxing and effective for people with tinnitus.

You can also buy a cassette or CD of soothing music from RNID or send off for a list of suggested recordings from the BTA. Hush also produces a relaxing seashore tape. (See *Chapter seven* for contact details).

Relaxation/stress therapy

A regular relaxation routine is a very helpful part of tinnitus management and can help you manage the stress that is often associated with tinnitus.

What has stress got to do with tinnitus?

Many people notice their tinnitus more when they are worried or tired, and this in turn increases their levels of anxiety and stress. This becomes a vicious circle. It is now widely accepted that stress plays a key part in the way people react to their tinnitus.

A certain amount of stress is vital to maintain the systems that alert us to possible dangers – for instance, those signals that tell us to leap out of the way of an oncoming car. However, in today's busy lifestyles there is a build up of 'stressors' – things that cause you intense pressure, tension or anxiety – which put both your body and mind on constant alert. You probably do not have enough time to relax and feel calm, so allowing your body and mind to rest. People react differently to different 'stressors', but your reactions to stress will happen whether you think about them or not.

What can be done about stress?

You can learn to control your responses to stress by using relaxation techniques. These are taught in many tinnitus clinics and audiology departments. You will also find local adult education classes teaching relaxation techniques, or you could try classes in meditation or yoga, for example, which can help you learn to relax. You can also buy guided relaxation cassettes and CDs from the RNID Tinnitus Helpline, or your local library may have some you can borrow.

Relaxation techniques can vary widely. They can include brief, 'time-out' exercises, which you can use if you are faced with a stressful event or as part of your everyday routine, or extended body and mind exercises, which create a sense of deep and total relaxation. These are usually practised lying down, in quiet, peaceful surroundings.

Exercises can be physical, for example, tensing and releasing your muscles, or psychological – where you use your imagination to help you relax. Some form of breathing exercise is usually a key part of a relaxation routine.

Being able to relax deeply is a skill and like anything else it takes time and effort to acquire that skill. But once you have learned to relax, it can help to break down the vicious cycle of listening to tinnitus and feeling stressed. This can help you get rid of feelings of distress and helplessness. It is also valuable in helping you keep a sense of good, general health and wellbeing. However, relaxation can only help if you learn how to do it and practise it regularly, preferably every day. If you don't do it, it can't work. You may find it helpful to practise with a partner.

Complementary medicines can also be useful to help control stress and so help you manage your tinnitus. We tell you more about these in *Chapter five*.

Counselling

Counselling is a very important part of all tinnitus management. It can enable you to understand your tinnitus. This helps you move forward and learn to habituate to it. Talking about your tinnitus and sharing how it makes you feel can also be very helpful.

Counselling for tinnitus may involve:

- Explaining what might be causing tinnitus.
- Helping you to understand that tinnitus is not a threat in any way.
- Correcting any false or unhelpful ideas about tinnitus.
- Helping you to identify and change behaviour and thoughts that may be tuning your sound response systems to tinnitus.
- Providing information about tinnitus.
- Suggesting ways of managing tinnitus.
- Demonstrating how to use a sound generator, sound enrichment or hearing aid.
- Teaching relaxation exercises.
- Helping you develop a positive attitude.
- Giving you support if you find tinnitus particularly troublesome.

A relaxation technique to try yourself

The following short technique can be helpful as part of a tinnitus management plan if you practise it regularly.

Before you begin

Turn off the television, unplug the telephone/textphone and lock your door if you think you may be disturbed.

Make yourself as comfortable as possible, preferably lying down, but if you are sitting in a chair make sure you are supported at the back and head – put your chair against a wall or use a high backed chair. Make sure you are warm enough because as you relax your body temperature may drop a little.

Play a calming and relaxing CD or cassette of music. Alternatively, use a tinnitus sound enricher and set the timer. If you find it difficult to listen to music because of your hearing loss, then use your other senses. Buy a relaxing herb pillow or use a room fragrance or scented candle. **Never fall asleep with a lighted candle and do not leave a lighted candle unattended**. Look at a peaceful and serene picture before you close your eyes and remember the image. Have something comforting to hold and feel.

The next few minutes are for you, they are as much a part of your healthcare as a prescription from your GP.

Close your eyes and enjoy...

Take a slow, deep breath, in through the nose, if possible, filling the lungs. Hold the breath for a moment, then breathe out slowly through your mouth.

- Repeat two to three times.

- Then breathe slowly and regularly throughout the exercise.

- Concentrate on your feet. In your mind tell them to feel calm, let them drop apart (if lying down). Let them become loose and floppy. Be aware of your feet, see them in your mind resting on the bed or floor.

- Then think about your calves, tell your muscles to relax, to let go and feel free.

- Next think about your thighs, tell your muscles to feel calm and at ease, be aware of the weight of your legs pressing on the surface they are resting on.

- Continue in this way, concentrating on each part of your body, think about each part in turn, and see a picture in your mind's eye – buttocks, stomach, back, arms, hands, shoulders, neck, head and face. Be aware of the difference between feeling tense and feeling relaxed.

- Enjoy this relaxed and calm feeling for a few minutes, listen to the music, or enjoy the scent of the room, let your thoughts come and go easily.

- After a few minutes, when you feel ready, start to be aware of the sounds around you, open your eyes and look around. Slowly and calmly sit up. Become alert and ready to carry on with the rest of your day, but keep with you your feelings of being calm, relaxed and at ease.

Tinnitus retraining therapy (TRT)

Some tinnitus clinics use tinnitus retraining therapy (TRT) which has been developed by Pawel Jastreboff and Jonathan Hazell. Anyone who provides TRT will have been specifically trained in how to use it. TRT uses a combination of sound therapy and directive counselling according to an individual management plan. Before treatment you will be carefully assessed, and the most effective treatment discussed with you. Some people only need one or two sessions, whilst others benefit from several months of treatment. TRT helps you habituate to your tinnitus, and you will be given a series of habituation exercises to use at home. TRT works by retraining the brain's sound response systems and the way your 'filters' tune in to tinnitus until you are eventually less aware of it and don't have a problem with it when you hear it.

Neurophysiologically based management

Most tinnitus clinics use a form of tinnitus management called neurophysiologically based management. This uses the basic concepts of TRT but in a less strictly controlled way and is usually very successful.

Cognitive behavioural therapy

Cognitive behavioural therapy is a technique used by some psychologists or psychotherapists. It is based on the idea that what we think affects how we behave. Cognitive behavioural therapy aims to find out what lies behind the way we behave and to change how we react to different situations. People can be very distressed by tinnitus because of what they believe about it. Sometimes these beliefs are not true. If beliefs about tinnitus are changed, the unpleasant feelings it produces can also be changed. Cognitive behavioural therapy also makes use of relaxation techniques and problem solving skills. By changing how you think about tinnitus and how you behave, you can reduce your distress and start to tolerate the noises you hear until eventually you notice them less.

Food and drink

No food or drink causes tinnitus. However, occasionally some people feel that certain foods and drinks alter the level of their tinnitus. The most common ones most people mention are:

- Caffeine – tea, coffee, chocolate, cola.
- Alcohol – especially red wine.
- Tobacco.
- Oranges, lemons, grapefruits.
- Spicy food – especially monosodium glutamate.
- Salt.

Do not give all of these up at once. If the tinnitus becomes quieter, you will never know what it was that made the difference! Only give up one thing at a time for a set period, say three weeks. If there is a difference, you may want to cut that food or drink out for longer. However, be sensible – if you enjoy these things, giving them up can make you resent your tinnitus.

It is a good idea to follow your GP or audiologist's advice if they suggest you give up a particular food or drink.

Sometimes tinnitus can appear to be louder first thing in the morning. There is some debate as to why this happens. Some researchers suggest that everyone's brain runs a quick 'security scan' on waking which, among other things, turns the hearing sensitivity to maximum. If you have tinnitus this makes it seem louder. Other researchers suggest that it may be due to low glucose levels, because you have not been eating whilst asleep.

Some researchers believe that the comforting routine of having a hot drink to start the day can relax and reassure you and so lowers the tinnitus. Others think that once you have got up in the morning you are more distracted so you don't think about the tinnitus so much.

Medication

If you feel that your medication may be affecting the tinnitus, discuss this with your GP. They may advise you to continue with your medication because the benefits are essential, or they may say that the dosage you are on is too low to have any effect on the tinnitus, or they may agree that the medicine is affecting the tinnitus, and change it.

You should *not* alter the dose of any medication you are taking, or stop taking it as a result of reading this book, unless the GP who prescribed the medication agrees it is safe to do so. If you have any questions about any medication you are taking, or are about to take, speak to your GP or pharmacist.

You will find more detailed information about drugs and tinnitus in *Chapter one*.

Managing tinnitus if you are severely or profoundly deaf

If you are severely or profoundly deaf, staff at your ENT department will be able to discuss the options available to help you manage tinnitus. These could include counselling, relaxation therapy, TRT, neurophysiologically based management and cognitive behavioural therapy.

You may like to try learning relaxation exercises from a book or class or see whether complementary therapies can help you relax and sleep. We have included a simple relaxation exercise earlier in this chapter. You can also discuss any medication you are taking with your GP. It is also important to get a good night's sleep. You should also make the most of any support available from friends, family or support groups. We look at these options in later chapters.

Can cochlear implants help tinnitus?

People using cochlear implants often find that their tinnitus is reduced or less noticeable. However, a small proportion of people report that the implant makes their tinnitus worse. It is important to get advice about this when you are being assessed for an implant.

Cochlear implants give a 'sensation' of hearing to severely or profoundly deaf adults and children. A cochlear implant is an electronic device that is made up of two parts. The external part is worn like a hearing aid, either on the head or clipped to clothes, and the internal part is surgically implanted in the ear. They are only provided via specialist centres in the UK.

Who are they suitable for?

Cochlear implants are not suitable for the vast majority of people with a hearing loss. They are only suitable for a few people who have profound sensorineural deafness in both ears, and who get little or no benefit from conventional hearing aids in both ears. Implants are suitable for some, but not all, adults who have become profoundly deaf after they have acquired spoken language skills. They are rarely considered suitable for adults who have been deaf from birth, or before learning to speak or understand language. This is because an adult needs some memory of sound in order to make sense of the signals passed to their brain by the implant. An implant may also be suitable for some deaf children. Anyone who is being considered for an implant will go through a rigorous selection and counselling process.

You can find out more from the RNID Tinnitus Helpline or the British Cochlear Implant Group (see *Chapter seven* for contact details).

Think positive!

None of the suggestions in this book will help unless you are prepared to put them into practise. Tinnitus management is not something that someone does for you, but what you do for yourself. You cannot improve your tinnitus by just reading this book – you need to carry out the ideas it contains.

Peter's story

Peter is 59. He has a slight hearing loss in his right ear and tinnitus in both ears.

My tinnitus started in 1998, while I was in Malaysia, after a case of flu. I had also been taking quinine. My ears felt blocked. I went to my GP on returning home and he recommended a spray, which I found impossible to use and which didn't work. I am grateful, though, that he sent me to see a specialist who referred me to a hearing therapist.

My family are very supportive, but I don't think anyone really understands what tinnitus is like unless they have it.

I didn't think there was much point in coming to see the hearing therapist unless I was prepared to try what she suggested, so I tried everything, but nothing was as effective as the white noise generator*. I wore it constantly for six hours a day, every day. I divided the six hours up into three lots of two hours. The tinnitus decreased very quickly and disappeared altogether during a trip to the Commonwealth Games. When the tinnitus returns occasionally, I just use the white noise generator again. It can be just as annoying sometimes as it was at first, but now I know it can be controlled.

*Also known as a sound generator.

Pauline's story

Pauline is 60. She has a mild hearing loss in both ears.

Well, my tinnitus started about two and a half years ago. My Mum died and then my Dad died ten months later. It was really bad when my Mum died. I had a really stressful time. The tinnitus is like a bee buzzing in my left ear and is worse when it's quiet. I was ever so frightened at first because I had heard of tinnitus. My Dad had it and he had it really badly but he wouldn't do anything about it. He wouldn't even wear his hearing aid. I didn't want to end up like him.

I went to my doctor about this tinnitus noise and he referred me to ENT and they recommended me to come to the tinnitus clinic. My GP was very helpful and as soon as he heard what the problem was he referred me at once. My hearing loss is not such a problem. I can't hear if someone speaks when they are behind me and sometimes I can't hear the doorbell. I don't like loud music. It seems to grate on my ears. I try to keep away from loud music at parties. I hate anything in my ears.

My husband is very good and so are my family. Until it happens to them, though, people don't really know what the noise is like and what you go through.

The hearing therapist made lots of suggestions but the one which really helped me was the CDs. I got in touch with the BTA and was sent their catalogue of tinnitus tapes and CDs. I find those mood CDs very helpful, especially the water sounds and things like that. They're nice when you come in from work. I listen to them quite a lot every day. I've even got a CD player in the bedroom. I listen to them for a long time. Even my husband's been listening to them.

My tinnitus is much better now. I don't hear it all when I'm busy. It doesn't bother me any more. I've got my life back.

Chapter four
A good night's sleep

This chapter looks at the importance of sleep and the link between sleep and tinnitus. It also gives you lots of practical advice to help you get a good night's sleep.

What is sleep and why do we need so much of it?

It is a sobering thought that anyone who lives to be at least 75 years old and who sleeps eight hours a night will spend approximately 220,000 hours of their life asleep! As you spend about one-third of your life sleeping you can see why it is important.

There is still a lot of debate about why we sleep. Some suggestions have included:

- Rest – from tiredness.
- Replenishing cells – growth.
- Restoration – healing.
- Resolving issues by dreaming about them – psychology.
- Recharging the brain cells – memory.
- Relief – from stress.

We cannot live without sleep and it is vital to our existence. The natural world has a 24-hour rhythm of light and darkness and we have a body clock that responds to this – we know it is time to go to bed even if we cannot see the sun. This natural rhythm is called circadian rhythm.

Some myths about sleep

I haven't slept for a week

Wrong. It is impossible not to sleep. You may not have been aware of falling asleep, but you will have slept for short periods, perhaps without realising it.

Everyone must have eight hours sleep a night

Wrong. We sleep less as we get older – this is completely normal. Different people need different amounts of sleep. You may only need six hours a night, in which case spending eight hours in bed trying to sleep is a waste of time.

I shouldn't wake during the night

Wrong. The older you get, the more likely you are to wake up during the night. Often you just turn over and go back to sleep again but sometimes you might get up and visit the bathroom or have a drink of water. Occasionally you might be woken by a noise in the street, maybe a car starting up, which has gone by the time you are fully awake.

Alcohol helps you sleep

Wrong. Alcohol does not help you sleep – in fact, it has the opposite effect. By disrupting the sleep pattern it can cause people to wake earlier and to lie awake for longer.

Tinnitus and sleep

So, what is the relationship between tinnitus and sleep? When people with tinnitus were asked by researchers to name the things that irritated them most about tinnitus, the majority of them mentioned that it interfered with a good night's sleep.

You may have noticed that tinnitus appears to be louder at night. This is because your bedroom is probably the nearest thing you have to a soundproof room in your house. It is quiet and dark, and while you are lying in bed you have nothing else to think about, except the fact that you are not asleep. Tinnitus is not necessarily louder at night, it just appears to be because there are no other sounds to compete with it.

Tinnitus will not wake you up at night, but if you do wake up, instead of turning over and going back to sleep you may tune into it. This can make it difficult to get back to sleep. It's not the tinnitus that has woken you up, even though it may seem like it because it is the first thing you notice as soon as you wake up.

How to get a good night's sleep

Many of these suggestions will sound like commonsense. The most important thing about commonsense is that it is fairly uncommon! Sleeping well is a habit and it is possible to learn good habits and unlearn bad ones in time.

Before bedtime

Fresh air and exercise are good for you and can help you to get a good night's sleep. However, it is important to exercise during the day and not during the evening near to bedtime. Exercise near bedtime will stimulate you and keep you awake.

If you want to sleep at night, do not sleep during the day. 'Resting the eyes' after lunch counts as sleeping too! If you feel sleepy during the day, occupy your mind or body, do not sit in a chair and let your mind wander – you will be asleep before you know it.

A healthy diet is essential for a healthy life. Your main meal of the day should not be eaten near bedtime. Food is fuel for the body and will give you energy. If you eat, your body thinks you are going to use all that energy and becomes alert and ready for action. Eat early in the evening and not late at night.

Tea, coffee, cola drinks and chocolate all contain caffeine. Caffeine is a stimulant, which will keep you awake. Try these suggestions:

- Drink tea and coffee during the day, but avoid it at bedtime.
- Drink decaffeinated tea and coffee only.
- Give up tea and coffee and try something else such as herbal tea.

If you have chronic pain, it is sensible to take some of your painkillers at bedtime so that the pain will not prevent you sleeping. **Always consult your GP about taking regular painkillers and do not exceed the stated dose. Remember that misuse of some painkillers can cause pain and can be dangerous.**

Bedtime

Humans are creatures of habit. We like habits – they make us feel secure and relaxed. Develop some bedtime habits. Doing the same thing every night prepares you for sleep. It sends messages to the brain saying, in effect, 'sleep'. You could try:

- Folding and putting away your clothes.
- Having a bath.
- Having a milk drink. Milk encourages sleep.
- Spraying your bedroom with lavender or sandalwood scented room spray.

Go to bed when you feel sleepy but get up at the same time every day. Do not 'sleep in'.

The bedroom

Your bed should be comfortable. If your mattress is over ten years old, the chances are that it needs replacing. Make sure you have the right number of pillows. Some people have found that altering the number of pillows they use changes the position of their head and neck, and this improves their tinnitus.

Try some lavender in your bedroom in the form of a pillow, bag, bar of soap, scented candle, room spray, or bowl of fresh lavender. Lavender is said to be calming and relaxing. **If you use a scented candle never leave it unattended or burning when you go to sleep.**

The room should not be hot and airless. If you can, leave a small window open a little. It is easier for most people to sleep in the dark, so make sure your curtains are good thick ones (or lined).

Do not use the bedroom to watch television or to do your accounts, as you will eventually come to associate the bedroom with staying awake rather than going to sleep.

Avoid the soundproof room effect. Some people's tinnitus appears louder in silence, so the sensible thing to do is to arrange for some noise in your bedroom. Popular and helpful sounds include:

- A ticking clock.
- An electric fan.
- A pillow speaker.
- A bedside sound generator.
- A sound pillow.
- Relaxing cassettes or CDs.
- A sound enricher. Some of the more recent models contain crystals that produce pleasant and relaxing smells.
- A small indoor water feature.

Do not use earplugs. They cut out external noise, can make tinnitus seem worse and are not usually helpful.

What if I wake up?

If you wake up and find it difficult to get back to sleep, don't lie awake worrying about being awake. The more you lie there thinking about how you cannot sleep, the more agitated you will become. The more agitated you become, the more difficult it is to sleep. Thinking about not sleeping can create a vicious circle. If you can't sleep, get up and find something to do. Wrap up warmly and sit in a chair. Try making a milk drink, reading, doing a crossword or writing a letter.

When you are sleepy, go back to bed. If you are still awake after 20 minutes, get up and repeat the procedure. Do not lie-in in the morning but get up at your usual time. Go to bed the following night when you feel sleepy.

Tips for dropping off to sleep

- Repeat a nonsense word.

- Count backwards – in threes!

- Remember the happiest day of your life.

- Don't go to sleep with a 'busy brain'.

- Try and put your problems aside to be dealt with another time. If you are worrying about a problem, keep a pad and pen by the bed and jot down the problem and what you could do about it. You will not necessarily solve the problem – some problems are hard to solve – but working through it may stop you worrying and help you to go to sleep.

- Remember, things always seem worse at night than in the morning.

- Try a relaxation technique. This can help you unwind and fall asleep. Visualisation and breathing exercises can be particularly helpful. See *Chapter three* for information about learning to relax.

Getting help from your GP

If you feel you need more help with your sleep, do ask your GP for advice.

Grace's story

Grace is 67. She has a mild hearing loss in both ears and tinnitus in her left ear.

I've had a lot of trouble with my ears over the years. I had this dreadful itching and pain in my left ear. The pain was so bad I couldn't rest my head on the pillow. My husband brought me up to casualty and the doctor said that the itching was caused by dead skin in my ear and the pain was caused by an infection. He gave me drops for the itching and antibiotics. I was told to see my GP. My GP sent me to the ENT clinic where I had my ear cleaned out. They also checked my throat and found that I had enlarged tonsils. I thought, at my age, I didn't want to have them out but the consultant assured me I would be safe. He did the operation himself and it was a great success. I was so pleased that I'd had them out and I felt much better.

Several months later I started getting this noise. I worried and worried. My husband worried too. He is not a well man and I had been worried about him. He said, "go and get an appointment to see somebody about that noise". I phoned the hospital and made an appointment to come to the clinic again. I was very worried. Some people at work had had tinnitus and they had said such things about it that I became quite frightened. I used to work in a very noisy factory and people in noisy factories sometimes get tinnitus. They really scared me.

I came to the tinnitus clinic and they were very helpful. They told me what to do. I drink decaffeinated coffee, listen to the radio and keep busy. My husband and I eat and drink the same things so we help each other stick to our diets.

I sleep well now. I only hear the tinnitus when I have to get up in the night to go to the toilet but I soon go back to sleep again. I know what's good for tinnitus and what's not good. I'm not worried about it any more. I'm OK.

Chapter five
Complementary medicine

Nowadays many people do try complementary medicine (sometimes known as alternative therapies) as a way of managing their own health needs. This chapter gives you some tips if you are thinking of trying complementary medicine for tinnitus and looks in more detail at some of the more common types of complementary medicine available.

Before you begin any course of complementary medicine it is always worth seeking conventional help for your tinnitus as you will be referred to experts who can explore your condition in full. Having done this, some people find it helpful to look at complementary medicine as well.

How can complementary medicine help tinnitus?

Broadly speaking, complementary therapies do not treat tinnitus as such, but they do offer a way to give you a sense of wellbeing. They can encourage your mind and body to unwind and help create a full, but calm and less stressful lifestyle. This has a 'knock-on' effect on tinnitus. It is important to realise that there is very little conclusive evidence to prove or disprove the usefulness of any particular complementary medicine. Most evidence is anecdotal (word of mouth). One theory is that they work by helping you to relax and sleep. Different therapies suit different people so it is a case of try it and see. If it works for you, use it, but be wary of leaping from one type to another in the hope of finding the 'miracle cure'. Complementary medicine can also take time to work and may not have an instant effect on your tinnitus, if at all.

Is complementary medicine available on the NHS?

Although complementary medicines are now much more widely recognised as a key part of modern medicine, they are not widely available on the NHS so can end up costing you a lot of money. However some GPs and physiotherapists do offer complementary medicines such as massage, acupuncture and homeopathy. There are also specialist NHS homeopathic hospitals in some parts of the UK. It is always worth checking with your GP to see if they have training in any of the complementary medicines. However, a lot of complementary medicine is only available through private practice where you will have to pay for it.

Before you start complementary medicine

■ Always consult a GP before trying any complementary medicine, especially if you are already taking conventional medication.

■ **Never stop taking prescribed medication without discussing it with the doctor who prescribed it.**

■ If you are going to use complementary medicine you can buy over-the-counter, check any possible side effects it may have and its compatibility with any other medication you are taking. Just because you are buying it over-the-counter doesn't meant it won't be harmful. This is particularly important if you are going to try preparations such as St John's Wort or Ginko Biloba.

■ Always use a complementary medicine practitioner who is qualified and registered with the relevant professional body. See *Chapter seven* for details.

During your visit to a complementary therapist

- Discuss tinnitus with the complementary therapist and make sure they know about the condition and can offer help.

- Make sure the therapist takes your full medical history and is aware of other treatments you are taking.

- Discuss possible numbers of treatments, costs of each session and length of time involved.

- Check that the therapist has suitable insurance cover. They should be insured against accidental injury to you or to your property, whether you are on their premises or on private premises. They should also have public liability insurance.

Deciding what to choose

Below is a summary of some complementary medicines that are more widely available. It is not a complete list nor does it recommend these treatments above any others. These therapies have been chosen as it will probably be easier to find someone practising them in your area.

Acupuncture, acupressure, shiatsu

These are ancient therapies where practitioners believe that vital energy flows through different channels, or meridians, in the body. When this flow becomes interrupted you may become ill. Various parts of the body are thought to connect directly to certain points on the skin and stimulating these points corrects the flow of energy and returns the body to good health.

- In acupuncture (Chinese therapy), the tips of needles are inserted into these specific points on the skin.

- In acupressure, pressure or suction is applied to these points.

- Shiatsu (a Japanese word meaning finger pressure) uses the same technique but practitioners also use massage, diet and exercise.

Aromatherapy, reflexology and massage

These use a combination of massage and aromatic oils, which come from plants. The specially blended oils can be used in body massage, baths, room scents and steam inhalations. Massage combines the senses of touch and smell to stimulate your circulation and move the oils around your body. These therapies are used to treat a wide variety of health problems, from everyday aches, pains and headaches, to stress and anxiety.

Chiropractic and osteopathy

These treatments are based on manipulating, massaging and stretching the joints and muscles, particularly the spinal column. They are used mainly for treating arthritic and rheumatic conditions, whiplash or sports injuries, and their effects on the nervous system.

Herbalism

Chinese herbalism makes a diagnosis based on a patient's pattern of symptoms rather than a named disease. It is part of a holistic approach to treatment. Chinese herbs are prescribed as pills, powders, pastes, ointments, creams and lotions.

Western herbalism makes formulas from whole plant parts traditionally found in the west. These contain a mix of ingredients that create a 'synergy', which enhances the effectiveness of the medicine.

Homeopathy

This therapy uses natural medicine. A homeopath aims to find a remedy, which, in high doses, would cause the symptoms similar to those being experienced by the patient. The aim is to go with, rather than against, the body's own efforts to heal itself. This is based on the principle that symptoms are the body's defences and therefore need helping not suppressing. Medicines are prescribed in very dilute forms and given to patients to take themselves.

Claire's story

Claire is 41 and has Menière's disease*. Tinnitus is one of the symptoms of her condition.

When I first heard the tinnitus I was quite frightened because I didn't know what it was and I imagined all kinds of horrible things. My tinnitus sounds like a rustling noise, which is more noticeable at night when I get a whistling noise as well. It's worse when I'm tired or stressed, those things definitely play a part.

Just before an attack of Menière's the tinnitus is very high pitched. If I go back to bed and rest I can sometimes prevent an attack. The tinnitus is an early warning signal.

The first person I turned to was my GP. He thought I had an ear infection and gave me antibiotics. When they didn't work he sent me to see a specialist. My GP has been very helpful and encouraging. I've found the low salt diet very helpful for the Menière's disease. I've also found that it's very helpful to listen to what your body is telling you. You know when you have been overdoing it and when you are tired or stressed.

Relaxation tapes help. They have taught me controlled breathing and visualisation, you know, "imagine you're in a beautiful garden" or "imagine you're in a white bubble when nothing can harm you or hurt you". When you feel bad you can imagine you are safe in that bubble.

Sometimes the tinnitus drives me crazy when I try to go to sleep at night. Then I use the pillow speaker or the tape of sea sounds. They help soothe the tinnitus and help me get to sleep.

I also have acupuncture. I don't know if it helps my Menière's disease and tinnitus, but it gives me a nice calm feeling which helps me to cope better.

*We tell you more about Menière's disease in *Chapter one*.

Chapter six
Support networks

This chapter suggest ways you can get additional support and help from people who are not professionals. It looks particularly at self-help groups and gives some tips on how to start one if there isn't one in your area.

What is a tinnitus support network?

A support network could be an individual, group or organisation that can offer you time and understanding about your experience of tinnitus. As well as the professional support available from your GP, and ENT, audiology and hearing therapy staff at your hospital or tinnitus clinic, your support network might be made up of:

- Family and friends.
- Colleagues.
- Support groups.
- Self-help groups.
- Local and national organisations, charities and voluntary groups.

How can support networks help?

Talking to someone who is understanding and supportive, rather than someone who offers pity or expresses regret, can be enormously helpful and speed up the process of coming to terms with tinnitus.

Family, friends and colleagues can be a valuable source of support, so it is important to make sure they are aware of your tinnitus and how it makes you feel. Make sure they are as informed as you are about tinnitus, so they can support you as you learn to manage it. You may find it helpful if they come to appointments with you.

Getting support from a group

Generally, self-help and support groups are run by people who share a common interest. Both offer the same kind of support but they can be very different in the way they are set up.

■ Self-help groups are more likely to be run for, and by, the members of the group themselves. They may charge a small fee for membership (or no fee at all) and are non-profit making. Self-help groups provide information. They are not intended to be therapy groups.

■ Support groups are mainly led by professionals or paid staff who ultimately take responsibility for the management and organisation of the group.

Why get support from a group?

■ Being in a group gives you the opportunity to meet others who have similar experiences to you. Meeting other people with tinnitus will help you realise that you are not alone.

■ A group can help you become more aware of your own health needs, feel empowered and in control.

■ Talking to others gives you a chance to share relevant, up-to–date information, new research and coping strategies.

■ Going to a group can give you confidence and self-esteem as your own knowledge and understanding develops.

■ Sharing experiences can help you reduce stress, fears and anxieties.

■ You can make new friends and use your experience to help someone else.

However, not everyone finds group work helpful so don't worry if they're not for you. If you do like the idea of trying a support group, make sure the group you choose is supportive and helpful rather than a forum for people to complain. Also, with time, as your tinnitus gets better, you may find that you no longer need to go to a group and talk about it.

The Chase Mentinns support group is one of several across the UK for people who have Menière's disease and/or tinnitus. This particular group is open to patients at Chase Farm Hospital in North London. Here they talk about why they come to the group.

"I don't feel so alone."

"I know I'm not the only one."

"Ours isn't a visible problem and other people get so impatient with you. They don't think you have a problem."

"People who don't have tinnitus tell you not to worry and to forget about it. They have no idea."

"One of the advantages of the group is that we support each other."

"We laugh at things together."

"We enjoy a social time and raise money for good causes."

"We suggest solutions to each other. Trying decaffeinated tea was a good idea."

"This morning I was glad I was coming here, I was really looking forward to it."

"At the group you find a friend to listen. Having tinnitus can be very lonely because no one wants to know."

"Other people ask how you are but they don't really want to know but people in the group really care and are interested."

"I think people have progressed since being in the group."

"Coming to the support group has improved my confidence."

Choosing a self-help group

Remember, self-help groups do not suit everybody. Some people find that being with other people who have similar health needs is quite distressing. However, the benefits can be invaluable for many people.

There are many organisations that can put you in touch with an established group. Try:

- The British Tinnitus Association.
- RNID Tinnitus Helpline.
- NHS Direct.
- The Menière's Society.
- The Internet.

Asking in your local library, GP surgery, or audiology or ENT department at your local hospital, for details of local groups.

What if there isn't a local group?

Start one! There is plenty of information available, offering good tips on how to do this. If you are interested try:

- Contacting other self-help groups in your local area to see how they did it.
- Contacting your local Council for Voluntary Service. Telephone numbers are listed in the telephone directory but if you need more help contact NACVS.
- Get in touch with Self Help Nottingham.

Claire's story

Claire, who has Menière's disease, talks about the support she gets from her local support group.

I'm very active in my local support group. I'm young and motivated and I've got access to the Internet so I feel it's up to me to make a positive contribution to the group. I think you get out what you put in.

You share experiences with other people in the group and exchange information. I've picked up things from other people. For example, I've got to go for some balance tests and a member of the group sent me a load of information and leaflets about them. You share views. Family and friends don't fully understand because they haven't got it. There are people in the group who have it worse – but they can cope so I know I will. You get reassurance and peace of mind.

The group is starting to gel. People are coming out of their shells and barriers are coming down all the time. At first everyone was very reserved and careful what they said. The same people come all the time so we can support each other and move forward.

Getting speakers in helps and makes the meetings interesting. So far we've had a hearing therapist and a dietician. Next meeting we're having someone from a carer's association and in the summer, someone from the Menière's Society. The two hearing therapists from the hospital come to the meeting as well.

The local newspaper is interested in doing an article on Menière's disease, tinnitus and our self-help group. I think this could be very helpful. It would let people know they're not alone and that our group is there to support them.

Getting started

Once you have decided to start a self-help group try to find two to three other people with tinnitus who are interested in helping you start a group. You can pool your skills, share ideas and create an action plan. You might like to think about:

- Getting help and advice from your local audiology department or tinnitus clinic.
- Whether you need to develop an existing group rather than setting up a new one.
- Getting as much information as possible from tinnitus organisations such as the British Tinnitus Association or the RNID Tinnitus Helpline, and from libraries and the Internet.
- Visiting other self-help groups (not necessarily tinnitus groups), to see how they did it.
- Advertising your group in the local newsagent, audiology department or GP surgery. Don't give your own personal details at this stage. A contact number may be sufficient.
- Where you will meet – in a member's home, village hall, scout hut or school hall. There could be costs involved.
- What area you will cover. This is important when thinking about advertising and travelling.
- How regularly the group will meet, membership fees, speakers and topics of interest.
- Confidentiality and respecting what other people need from the group.
- Establishing the group's boundaries, for example, who can join, will carers be invited, can people with an associated condition, for example Menière's disease, be included?
- Whether you have the time and energy to set up a group?
- What will the effect be on family and friends and your social life?
- Whether there are enough people to share the work?

Most of all you should enjoy setting up and taking part in the group. Self-help is literally what it says – do-it-yourself – but it is also about mutual help. Most people find that they get out as much as they put in – everyone helps each other! Support from professionals is there if you need it but this is an opportunity to do it your way.

Remember, coping with other people's difficulties can be emotionally draining. Guard against too much negativity, the aim should be positive support. You do not want to increase your own stress levels!

See *Chapter seven* for contact details for all organisations mentioned in this chapter.

Further information

Help and advice about tinnitus

RNID Tinnitus Helpline

The RNID Tinnitus Helpline offers information and advice to people with tinnitus, their families and friends and the professionals who work with them. We can put you in touch with your nearest self-help group. We also publish factsheets and leaflets and a newsletter – *Tinnitus Focus* – and sell a range of CDs and cassettes to help you relax.

RNID Tinnitus Helpline, 19-23 Featherstone Street,
London EC1Y 8SL
Tel: 0808 808 6666
Textphone: 0808 808 0007
Fax: 020 7296 8199
E-mail: tinnitushelpline@rnid.org.uk
Website: www.rnid.org.uk

British Tinnitus Association (BTA)

The British Tinnitus Association campaigns for better services for people with tinnitus. It supports a network of local tinnitus groups around the country, has a range of publications and produces a quarterly magazine – *Quiet*. You can also contact British Tinnitus Association for details of CDs and cassettes to help you relax.

British Tinnitus Association, Ground Floor, Unit 5, Acorn Business Park, Woodseats Close, Sheffield S8 0TB
Tel: 0800 018 0527
Fax: 0114 258 7059
E-mail: info@tinnitus.org.uk
Website: www.tinnitus.org.uk

Information about tinnitus on the Internet

RNID takes no responsibility for the contents of other websites, nor can it be responsible for any of the materials or postings on any of the Internet chatrooms. If you are unhappy with the content of any of the sites listed below, please direct your inquiries or complaints to the company hosting the site.

www.ata.org
The American Tinnitus Association's website.

www.tinnitus.asn.au
The Australian Tinnitus Association's website.

www.iths.net
The International Tinnitus and Hyperacusis Society promotes basic and clinical research in the areas of tinnitus, hyperacusis, and other closely related topics.

www.tinnitusbham.org.uk
The website for the Birmingham and District Tinnitus Group.

www.tinnitusexplained.org
The website for Hush, the Hull tinnitus self-help group. They sell a seashore tape for people with tinnitus.

www.tinnitus.org
The Tinnitus and Hyperacusis Centre's website. It gives information about tinnitus (and hyperacusis) retraining therapy.

www.tinnitus-pjj.com
The website for Jastreboff's Tinnitus and Hyperacusis centre.

Special equipment to help manage your tinnitus

You can buy sound pillows, sound generators and sound enrichers from a range of manufacturers and suppliers. Contact the RNID Tinnitus Helpline for an up-to-date list. RNID Sound Advantage also sells a range of products for people with tinnitus.

RNID Sound Advantage

You can visit the RNID Shop at www.rnidshop.com to buy equipment for deaf and hard of hearing people and people with tinnitus. Alternatively, send off for a copy of the RNID Sound Advantage *Solutions* catalogue.

RNID Sound Advantage, 1 Haddonbrook Business Centre, Orton Southgate, Peterborough PE2 6YX
Tel: 01733 232607
Textphone: 01733 238020
Fax: 01733 361161
E-mail: solutions@rnid.org.uk
Website: www.rnidshop.com

Further information about deafness and hearing loss

Defeating Deafness

The Defeating Deafness Information Service has up-to-date information on the latest advances in health care and research in the fields of hearing loss and tinnitus.

Defeating Deafness, The Hearing Research Trust, 330-332 Gray's Inn Road, London WC1X 8EE
Tel: 0808 808 2222
Textphone: 020 7915 1412
Fax: 020 7278 0404
Email: ddeafness.info@ucl.ac.uk
Website: www.defeatingdeafness.org

The National Deaf Children's Society (NDCS)
NDCS supports deaf children, young deaf people and their families in overcoming the challenges of childhood deafness.

The National Deaf Children's Society, 15 Dufferin Street,
London EC1Y 8UR
Tel: 0808 800 8880
Textphone: 0808 800 8880
Fax: 020 7251 5020
E-mail: helpline@ndcs.org.uk
Website: www.ndcs.org.uk

RNID Information Line
The RNID Information Line offers a wide range of information on many aspects of deafness and hearing loss. We also have a wide range of information factsheets and leaflets.

RNID Information Line, 19-23 Featherstone Street,
London EC1Y 8SL
Tel: 0808 808 0123
Textphone: 0808 808 9000
Fax: 020 7296 8199
E-mail: informationline@rnid.org.uk
Website: www.rnid.org.uk

Forest Books
A bookshop specialising in books about deafness and hearing loss.

Forest Bookshop Warehouse, Unit 2, New Building, Ellwood Road, Milkwall, Coleford, Gloucestershire GL16 7LE
Tel: 01594 833858.
Textphone: 01594 833507
Videophone: 01594 810637
Fax: 01594 833446
E-mail: forest@forestbooks.com
Website: www.forestbooks.com

General health information and advice

Medical Advisory Service

General advice about health including sleep problems.

Medical Advisory Service, PO Box 3087, London W4 4ZP
Tel: 0208 994 9874
Fax: 0208 995 3275

NHS Direct

Free health information on the Internet and over the tel/textphone.

Tel: 0845 4647
Textphone: 0845 606 46 47
Website: www.nhsdirect.nhs.uk

Menière's disease

The Menière's Society

The Menière's Society can provide information on all aspects of Menière's disease and can advise and support people with Menière's disease, and their families.

The Menière's Society, 98 Maybury Road, Woking GU21 5HX
Tel: 01483 740597
Textphone: 01483 771207
Fax: 01483 755441
E-mail: info@menieres.org.uk
Website: www.menieres.org.uk

Cochlear implants

British Cochlear Implant Group

The British Cochlear Implant Group represents all the cochlear implant centres and other specialist medical practitioners throughout the UK. Their website has been designed to provide information for medical professionals, people with cochlear implants, potential patients and their families.

Website: www.bcig.org

National Cochlear Implant Users Association (NCIUA)

NCIUA is a forum for cochlear implant users and their families.

NCIUA, PO Box 260, High Wycombe, Bucks HP11 1FA
Fax: 01494 484993
E-mail: jeriches@waitrose.com
Website: www.nciua.demon.co.uk

Complementary medicines

British Complementary Medicine Association

Can put you in touch with professional bodies to help you find a qualified practitioner.

British Complementary Medicine Association, PO Box 5122,
Bournemouth, Dorset BH8 0WG
Tel: 0845 345 5977
Fax: 0845 345 5977
E-mail: info@bcma.co.uk
Website: www.bcma.co.uk

Institute for Complementary Medicine (ICM)

Contact the ICM if you would like to find a practitioner listed on the British Register of Complementary Medicine.

ICM, PO Box 194, London SE16 7QZ
Tel: 020 7237 5165
Fax: 020 7237 5175
E-mail: icm@icmedicine.co.uk
Website: www.icmedicine.co.uk

Setting up a self-help group

NACVS

A CVS is a voluntary organisation that supports, promotes and develops local voluntary and community action. Find your nearest CVS in the telephone directory or contact NACVS.

NACVS, Arundel Court, 177 Arundel Street, Sheffield S1 2NU
Tel: 0114 278 6636
Textphone: 0114 278 7025
Fax: 0114 278 7004
E-mail: nacvs@nacvs.org.uk
Website: www.nacvs.org.uk

Self Help Nottingham

A charity which encourages the development of self help groups.

Self Help Nottingham, Ormiston House, 32-36 Pelham Street, Nottingham NG1 2EG
Tel: 0115 911 1662
Textphone: 0115 911 1655
Fax: 0115 911 1660
E-mail: admin@selfhelp.org.uk
Website: www.selfhelp.org.uk

Further reading

Alexander J. *Mind, Body, Spirit: A Complete Guide to Holistic Therapies for Achieving and Maintaining Optimum Health and Wellbeing.* 2003. (Carlton Books).

Hallam R. *Living with tinnitus: Dealing with the Ringing in Your Ears.* 1993. (HarperCollins).

Henry J, Wilson P. *Tinnitus. A Self-management Guide for the Ringing in Your Ears.* 2002. (Allyn and Bacon).

Johnston F. *Getting a Good Night's Sleep.* 2000. (Sheldon Press).

Kellerhals B and Zogg R. *Tinnitus Rehabilitation by Retraining: A Workbook for Sufferers, Their Doctors and Other Health Care Professionals.* 1999. (Karger).

Lavery S. *The healing power of sleep: How to achieve restorative sleep naturally.* 1997. (Gaia Books Ltd).

Lewith G. *Understanding Complementary Medicine.* 2002. (British Medical Association, Family Doctor Publications).

Rees D and Smith S. *Living with Tinnitus.* 1991. (Manchester University Press).

Self Help Nottingham. *Starting off Pack: Information and ideas for new Self-Help groups.* 1994. (Self Help Nottingham).

Tinnitus CDs and cassettes

Recommended by people with tinnitus, RNID's range of CDs and cassettes have easy to follow relaxation exercises and/or soothing music for you to relax to.

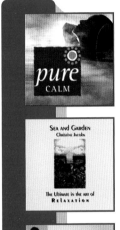

Pure Calm – relax as tranquil music helps you drift away from your every day problems.

Sea and Garden – a guided relaxation programme that takes you through two simple relaxation journeys.

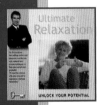

Ultimate Relaxation – TV Dr Hilary Jones talks about why we get stressed and guides you through practical exercises to help you relax.

For information please contact:

RNID Tinnitus Helpline
19-23 Featherstone Street
London EC1Y 8SL
Tel 0808 808 0666
Textphone 0808 808 0007
Fax 020 7296 8199
E-mail tinnitushelpline@rnid.org.uk
Website www.rnid.org.uk

Available now!

CDs
£11.99 each

Cassettes
£8.99 each

Contact **RNID**

for the latest information for deaf and
hard of hearing people and people with tinnitus

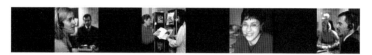

The **RNID** Tinnitus Helpline

If you have tinnitus, or work with people with tinnitus, we can give
you specialist information and advice.

RNID Tinnitus Helpline, 19-23 Featherstone Street,
London EC1Y 8SL
Tel 0808 808 6666
Textphone 0808 808 0007
Fax 020 7296 8199
E-mail tinnitushelpline@rnid.org.uk
Website www.rnid.org.uk

The **RNID** Information Line

The RNID Information Line is a great place to start if you want
information on many aspects of deafness or hearing loss, or
about the work we do.

RNID Information Line, 19-23 Featherstone Street,
London EC1Y 8SL.
Tel 0808 808 0123
Textphone 0808 808 9000
Fax 020 7296 8199
E-mail informationline@rnid.org.uk
Website www.rnid.org.uk

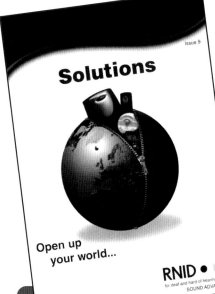

Become a **member**

The information and advice that you have received in this book does not stop here. Joining the other 34,000 RNID members is an excellent way of receiving up-to-date information on deafness, hearing loss and tinnitus as well as our influential campaigns. All members benefit from:

- **One in Seven**, our information packed bi-monthly magazine.

- **10% off** RNID priced publications.

- A **£5 voucher** towards equipment from RNID Sound Advantage.

- Access to **RNID Select** – special offers on a range of leading brands.

- Being part of the **campaign** to improve the lives of deaf and hard of hearing people.

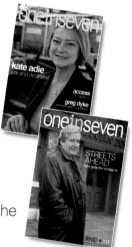

How to **join**

Membership is open to all and costs £19.50 per year, or only £12.50 if you are retired, unwaged or a full time student. It's easy to join:

Visit **www.rnid.org.uk/join** or

Call **020 7296 8049** (tel/textphone) for an application form.

You can save £2 off the standard price of membership by paying by Direct Debit. Contact the Membership Helpline on tel/textphone 020 7296 8049 for information.

Stay informed and **join today!**

RNIDtypetalk

Helping everyone
use the phone

Did you know, even if you have lost your hearing or your voice you can still use the telephone?

RNID Typetalk is the only national telephone relay service for deaf, deafened, deafblind, hard of hearing and speech-impaired people.

Making a call through RNID Typetalk is just like making a standard telephone call. You can have a full, real-time conversation, unlike SMS text messaging where you have to wait for the next part of the message.

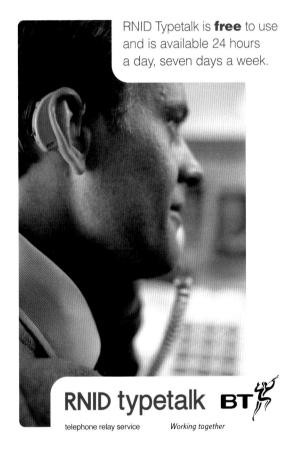

RNID Typetalk is **free** to use and is available 24 hours a day, seven days a week.

RNID typetalk **BT**
telephone relay service   *Working together*

For more information visit our website at **www.typetalk.org** or call our Customer Support Team free on:

Tel 0800 7311 888 **Textphone** 18001 0800 500 888
(Monday to Friday 8am-8pm. Weekends 9am-5pm)

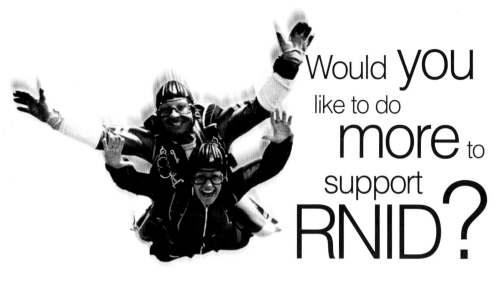

Would **you** like to do **more** to support RNID?

There are many ways you could help deaf and hard of hearing people in the UK, for example:

- Become a volunteer
- Make a donation
- Support our campaigns
- Take part in a sponsored challenge event
- Fundraise within your community
- Fundraise at work

For more information please contact

Supporter Services

Tel 020 7296 8399 **Textphone** 020 7296 8399

Fax 020 7296 8129 **E-mail** events@rnid.org.uk

It is only with the support of people like you that we can continue our vital work
Thank you!